WEIGHT LIFTING

A Beginner's Guide to
Progressive Weight Training, Workout Splits,
& Techniques

CALVIN PENNICK JR

This Page Left Blank Intentionally

Copyright

For permission requests, contact:
CPJR Publishing, Houston, Texas
www.cpjrpublishing.com

ISBN 979-8-9939686-1-2
Printed in the United States of America

Design and layout by Calvin Pennick JR

Disclaimer

This guide is for educational and informational purposes only. It is not intended as a substitute for professional medical advice, diagnosis, or treatment. Always consult your physician or other qualified health-care provider before beginning any exercise program, especially if you have a medical condition, are pregnant, or are taking medication. Stop any exercise that causes pain, dizziness, or shortness of breath and seek medical advice promptly.

Neither the author nor the publisher assumes any responsibility for injuries, losses, or damages that may result from following the information in this book.

Some portions of this guide were created or refined using artificial-intelligence tools under the author's supervision. All material has been carefully edited and fact-checked to ensure clarity, accuracy, and safety. AI assistance was used strictly as a creative and editorial aid, not as a source of medical or professional fitness instruction.

Contents

This Page Left Blank Intentionally

Introduction

Welcome to Weight Lifting: A Beginner's Guide to Weight Training Techniques, Workout Splits & Progression.

This book was written to simplify strength training for real people who want results without the confusion of conflicting fitness advice. Whether you train in a gym or at home, the concepts inside will help you build strength, confidence, and structure in your workouts.

You'll discover how to select the right workout split, master essential lifting techniques, apply progressive overload, and design programs that fit your lifestyle. Every section was written to build upon the last so that by the end of this guide, you'll not only know what to do—but why you're doing it.

If you've ever felt overwhelmed by workout plans or frustrated by slow progress, this book will give you the clarity and systems to train smarter, recover better, and see measurable results in as little as twelve weeks.

This Page Left Blank Intentionally

How to Use This Guide

This guide is designed as both a reference manual and a step-by-step roadmap:

1. Start with the Foundations – Read Sections 1–3 to understand workout splits, training methods, and how to match them to your goals and schedule.

2. Apply the Framework – Use Sections 4–7 to structure your own 12-week progression plan, adjusting intensity and volume as described.

3. Train with Purpose – Follow the sample workouts in Section 12. Track weights, reps, and effort (RPE/RIR) in a notebook or app.

4. Adapt as Needed – If you train at home, Section 8 shows how to modify each split using minimal equipment.

5. Support Recovery – Review Section 9 for nutrition, sleep, and lifestyle strategies to keep performance and recovery balanced.

6. Integrate Everything – Section 10 ties it all together into an actionable roadmap so you can maintain momentum long term.

Tip: Keep the guide open or printed near your training area. Revisit each section as your experience grows—what feels basic now will become invaluable when you're refining your own programs later.

Section 1:
What Is a Workout Split?

When you hear the phrase *"workout split,"* it simply refers to the way your training is **divided across the week**. Think of it as the blueprint that determines **which muscles you train, how often you train them, and how much recovery they get**. Choosing the right split is one of the most important decisions you'll make in structuring a fitness plan, because it directly shapes your results.

At its core, a workout split answers two key questions:

What body parts or movement patterns am I training today?

When will I train the others?

Splits are not just about organization — they are about **balancing stress and recovery**. Too much frequency and you risk over training. Too little frequency and progress slows. A well-chosen split aligns with your goals, lifestyle, and recovery ability.

Common Types of Splits

Full-Body Split
Every workout trains the entire body. This is ideal for beginners, time-crunched individuals, or anyone focusing on strength and skill development. Each muscle gets worked multiple times per week, which accelerates learning proper form.

Upper/Lower Split
One day targets the upper body, the next targets the lower body. This is popular with intermediate lifters because it balances training volume with recovery. It usually runs on a 4-day-per-week schedule.

Push/Pull/Legs (PPL)
This divides workouts into *pushing muscles* (chest, shoulders, triceps), *pulling muscles* (back, biceps), and *legs* (quads, hamstrings, glutes, calves). PPL is highly flexible and can be run as a 3-day plan (each once per week) or a 6-day plan (each done twice).

Body-Part Split

Also called a "bro split," this approach dedicates one day to one or two muscle groups (e.g., chest day, back day). It allows for very high volume on each muscle but requires 5–6 days in the gym for full coverage. Best for advanced lifters chasing maximum muscle size.

Why Splits Matter

The split you choose determines:

Frequency – How many times per week a muscle is trained.

Volume – How many total sets and reps per week for each muscle.

Recovery – How much rest a muscle gets before being worked again.

Focus – Whether the program emphasizes strength, hypertrophy, endurance, or conditioning.

In other words, the split is the **engine of your training program**. Without it, workouts become random and progress stalls.

Choosing the Right Split

If you're brand new or only have 2–3 days per week → start with a Full-Body Split.

If you're intermediate with 3–4 days available → go with Upper/Lower or PPL.

If you're advanced and highly committed (5–6 days) → choose PPL run twice per week or a Body-Part Split.

If you're time-crunched → focus on Full-Body or circuit-style training.

If you're concerned about joint health → prioritize TriCon or Tempo-based training within whichever split you choose.

Golden Rule: The best split isn't the one that looks "hardcore" on paper. It's the one you can **follow consistently, recover from, and progress on over time**.

Section 2:
Training Techniques

Once you've chosen your workout split, the next question becomes *"How should I train within each session?"* This is where training techniques come in. A training technique is simply a method for performing sets and reps to target specific outcomes such as **strength, size, endurance, or joint health**. Understanding the most popular techniques will give you more tools to shape your training around your goals.

Below are the most widely used and time-tested training techniques, with a focus on *what they are, why they're popular, and who they're best for.*

Progressive Overload

Definition: Gradually increasing the weight, reps, or sets over time to force the body to adapt.

Why It Works: It is the foundation of all strength and muscle growth. Without progressive overload, progress eventually stalls.

Best For: Everyone — beginners through advanced lifters.

Key Benefit: Scientifically proven pathway to continuous progress.

Main Limitation: Requires patience and consistency; results take time.

Compound Lifts

Definition: Multi-joint exercises like squats, deadlifts, bench presses, and pull-ups that recruit multiple muscles at once.

Why It Works: Builds the most strength and efficiency in the least amount of time. These lifts also carry over to real-life movement and athletics.

Best For: Strength development, athletic performance, and overall muscle building.

Key Benefit: Train multiple muscle groups at once; high efficiency.

Main Limitation: Technical lifts require excellent form to prevent injury; more taxing on the nervous system.

Isolation Training

Definition: Single-joint exercises like bicep curls, lateral raises, and leg extensions that target one muscle group.

Why It Works: Helps correct weak points, bring up lagging muscles, and sculpt physique details.

Best For: Bodybuilders, physique-focused trainees, or rehab purposes.

Key Benefit: Precise focus on one muscle group at a time.

Main Limitation: Limited carryover to overall strength; less efficient for calorie burn.

High-Intensity Training (HIT)

Definition: Short, intense workouts with sets taken very close to failure, often with minimal rest.

Why It Works: Maximizes effort in a short time and provides strong muscle stimulus.

Best For: People with limited time or those who prefer brief, intense sessions.

Key Benefit: Maximizes muscle recruitment in a short period.

Main Limitation: Can be mentally and physically exhausting; tough to sustain long term.

Supersets & Circuits

Definition: Performing two or more exercises back-to-back with little or no rest.

Why It Works: Increases training density, saves time, and boosts conditioning while still building muscle.

Best For: Fat loss, endurance, and general conditioning.

Key Benefit: Save time while keeping heart rate elevated.

Main Limitation: May reduce maximum strength performance if used too often.

Drop Sets

Definition: Perform a set to failure, reduce the weight by 20–30%, and immediately continue with more reps.

Why It Works: Extends time under tension and creates deep muscular fatigue, leading to hypertrophy.

Best For: Intermediate and advanced lifters focused on size.

Key Benefit: Extends sets beyond normal failure for a strong muscle-building stimulus.

Main Limitation: Highly fatiguing; recovery demands are significant.

Pyramid Training

Definition: Adjusting reps and weights each set, typically starting with lighter weights for higher reps and building up to heavier weights with lower reps.

Why It Works: Trains both muscular endurance and strength in a single workout.

Best For: Lifters seeking variety and balanced development.

Key Benefit: Trains multiple rep ranges in one session.

Main Limitation: Time-consuming; may cause fatigue before heavy sets.

Tempo Training

Definition: Controlling the speed of each rep, especially the lowering (eccentric) phase. For example, lowering a weight in 4 seconds instead of 1.

Why It Works: Increases time under tension and improves

mind-muscle connection.

Best For: Hypertrophy, joint-friendly training, and technical mastery.

Key Benefit: Improves mind-muscle connection and builds discipline under the bar.

Main Limitation: Mentally demanding; harder to track progress objectively.

TriCon Training

Definition: "Triple Contraction" — perform 3 explosive reps, 3 isometric holds, and 3 slow controlled reps in each set.

Why It Works: Builds muscle using lighter loads, making it easier on the joints while still creating intensity.

Best For: Lifters over 40, those with joint issues, or anyone wanting a different hypertrophy stimulus.

Key Benefit: Builds muscle without heavy weights; joint-friendly and unique.

Main Limitation: Less familiar; fewer resources and programs available.

Push/Pull/Legs (PPL) Structure

Definition: Not just a split, but also a technique of grouping muscles by movement pattern: push (chest, shoulders, triceps), pull (back, biceps), and legs.

Why It Works: Promotes balanced development and can be scaled from 3 to 6 days per week.

Best For: Intermediate to advanced trainees seeking flexibility and efficiency.

Key Benefit: Scales easily from 3 to 6 days per week, fits many goals.

Main Limitation: Works best if you can commit to at least 3 days per week; not ideal for those with very limited time.

Key Takeaway

Most lifters don't use just one technique. A well-rounded program blends **progressive overload with compound lifts** as the foundation, then layers in techniques like **drop sets, tempo, or TriCon** for variety and hypertrophy. The technique you emphasize should always align with your current goals and recovery ability.

Section 3: How to Choose a Workout Split

Choosing the right workout split is one of the most important steps in building a successful fitness program. A split is not just a schedule — it is the **framework that balances effort, recovery, and results**. The "best" split for you is the one that fits your **experience, goals, lifestyle, and recovery capacity**.

Let's break it down in detail.

Experience Level

Your training age — how long you've been lifting consistently — plays a huge role.

Beginners (0–1 year of consistent training)

Best Choice: Full-Body Split (2–3 sessions per week).

Why: Every muscle is trained multiple times per week, accelerating skill learning and strength development. Beginners don't need much volume per muscle group to see progress, so frequent practice with moderate weight is ideal.

Example: Monday, Wednesday, Friday → Squat, Bench, Deadlift variations + accessory work.

Intermediates (1–3 years)

Best Choice: Upper/Lower Split or Push/Pull/Legs (PPL).

Why: At this stage, you need more sets per muscle group to grow. Splitting the body into halves (Upper/Lower) or movement patterns (PPL) gives enough frequency while allowing recovery.

Example: 4-day Upper/Lower routine with 2 upper sessions and 2 lower sessions.

Advanced (3+ years)

Best Choice: PPL run twice weekly (6 days) or Body-Part Split.

Why: Advanced lifters require higher volume and intensity to continue progressing. These splits allow specialization — hammering one or two muscle groups with focused effort.

Example: A 6-day PPL: Push, Pull, Legs repeated twice, with varied intensity across the week.

Weekly Schedule & Lifestyle

Your available training days matter just as much as your experience.

2–3 Days Available: Full-Body Split or PPL once per week. Keeps things balanced without missed muscles.

3–4 Days Available: Upper/Lower or PPL. Both allow each muscle to be trained 1–2 times weekly.

5–6 Days Available: PPL (run twice) or Body-Part Split. Great for maximizing volume, aesthetics, and specialization.

Unpredictable/Busy Schedule: Full-Body is best, because even if you miss a day, you've still trained every muscle that week.

Rule of Thumb: Don't force a 6-day split if your life only allows 3 days. It's better to be consistent with fewer sessions than inconsistent with too many.

Training Goals

The split you choose should reflect what you're trying to achieve.

Strength: Choose Full-Body or Upper/Lower. They emphasize compound lifts (squat, bench, deadlift, overhead press) and allow heavier loads with more recovery.

Hypertrophy (muscle size): Choose PPL or Body-Part Split. They provide more volume per muscle group, include advanced techniques like drop sets and tempo, and allow focus on aesthetics.

Fat Loss & Conditioning: Supersets, Circuits, and HIT can be added to any split, but Full-Body and PPL tend to be most efficient for calorie burn and metabolic demand.

Joint Health & Longevity: Any split works, but use **Tempo Training** or **TriCon Training** to reduce joint strain while still stimulating growth.

Recovery Capacity

Your ability to recover — influenced by sleep, nutrition, age, and stress — dictates how much training you can handle.

High Recovery Capacity: Younger lifters, athletes, or those with low stress and good nutrition can often thrive on higher-frequency splits like PPL x2 or Body-Part Splits.

Moderate Recovery Capacity: Most people fall here. An Upper/Lower or 3–4 day PPL is often the sweet spot.

Low Recovery Capacity: Older lifters, those with injuries, or people under heavy work/life stress benefit more from Full-Body or low-frequency PPL (3 days/week).

Practical Guidelines for Choosing

Be Honest About Your Lifestyle: If you're a busy professional or parent, don't plan for 6 days in the gym. Choose something realistic.

Prioritize Consistency: The "best" split doesn't work if you can't stick to it.

Adjust Over Time: Start simple, then increase complexity as your experience and capacity grow. Many lifters begin with Full-Body, transition to Upper/Lower, and eventually try PPL or Body-Part Splits.

Test & Refine: If progress stalls or recovery feels inadequate, don't be afraid to adjust your split.

Bottom Line:
The right workout split is the one you can perform **consistently, recover from fully, and progress on steadily**. Instead of asking *"What's the hardest split?"* ask *"What split matches my life and allows me to train hard week after week?"*

This Page Left Blank Intentionally

Section 4:
Global Set, Rep & Effort Guidelines

No matter which split or training technique you use, the effectiveness of your program depends on **how you structure your sets, reps, intensity, and rest periods.** These variables determine whether you build strength, muscle, endurance, or simply burn calories. Understanding the science behind them ensures you train with purpose rather than guessing.

Rep Ranges and Their Purpose

Different rep ranges stimulate the body in different ways. While there is overlap, here's a useful breakdown:

Strength (1–6 reps):
Heavy weights for low reps build maximum force production. Think squats, deadlifts, and bench presses in the 3–5 rep range. Rest is longer to allow recovery of the nervous system.

Hypertrophy (6–12 reps, and up to 20–30 if near failure):
Moderate weight with moderate-to-high reps is best for muscle growth. This range provides a balance of mechanical tension (heavy load) and metabolic stress (the "burn" from higher reps). Studies show hypertrophy can happen anywhere from 6–30 reps if sets are taken close to failure.

Muscular Endurance / Conditioning (12–20+ reps):
Lighter loads with higher reps improve stamina and work capacity. Great for circuits, conditioning, and accessory exercises.

Key Point: Strength is best built with low reps, muscle growth with moderate reps, and endurance with high reps — but all three can overlap when effort is high.

Sets per Muscle Group

Volume (total sets per week per muscle group) is a major driver of progress.

Beginners: 6–10 sets per muscle group per week.

Intermediates: 10–15 sets per muscle group per week.

Advanced: 15–20+ sets per muscle group per week.

Example: If you bench press (4 sets), do incline dumbbell presses (4 sets), and dips (3 sets) in one week, that's **11 sets for chest**.

Rest Periods

Rest is often overlooked, but it determines whether you're ready to perform your next set effectively.

Strength Work (compounds, 4–6 reps): 2–4 minutes.

Hypertrophy (moderate isolation, 8–12 reps): 60–90 seconds.

Endurance/Conditioning (high reps, circuits, TriCon): 30–60 seconds.

Rule: Heavier lifts need more rest. Lighter, higher-rep work thrives on shorter rest to keep intensity high.

Intensity Tools: RPE and RIR

Two of the most useful tools for gauging effort are **RPE** and **RIR**. They help you train hard enough to progress without burning out.

RPE (Rate of Perceived Exertion): A 1–10 scale where 1 is "easy warm-up" and 10 is "all-out effort, no reps left."

> *RPE 6* = Comfortable, 4 reps left in the tank.
> *RPE 8* = Challenging, 2 reps left.
> *RPE 9* = Very challenging, 1 rep left.
> *RPE 10* = Maximum effort, failure.

RIR (Reps in Reserve): Counts how many reps you could have done before failure.

> *RIR 3* = You stopped with 3 reps left in the tank.
> *RIR 1* = You stopped with 1 rep left.
> *RIR 0* = You went to failure.

These scales connect: RPE 8 ≈ RIR 2.

How to Use Them:

Strength training should usually stay around **RPE 7–9 (1–3 RIR)**.

Hypertrophy sets are most effective at **RPE 8–9 (1–2 RIR)**.

Endurance and conditioning can safely push to **RPE 9–10 (0–1 RIR)** since the loads are lighter.

This helps you train hard enough to grow without maxing out every session, which leads to burnout or injury.

Effort Guidelines for Special Techniques

Drop Sets: Take the first set to near failure (RPE 9–10), then immediately reduce weight and continue.

Tempo Training: Keep RPE moderate (7–8), because slowing reps increases fatigue even with lighter weights.

TriCon Training: Typically performed at **RPE 8**, since the isometric holds and slow reps create huge tension without heavy weights.

Putting It Together

Strength Days: 4–6 sets, 4–6 reps, RPE 7–9, long rest.

Hypertrophy Days: 3–4 sets, 8–12 reps (or 12–20 on accessories), RPE 8–9, moderate rest.

Conditioning Days: 3–5 rounds, 10–20 reps, RPE 9–10, short rest.

TriCon Blocks: 3 sets of 9 reps (triple contraction), RPE 8, rest 90 seconds.

Bottom Line: You don't need to guess. Use rep ranges to match your goals, track weekly sets to ensure enough volume, rest appropriately between sets, and use RPE/RIR to regulate intensity. Train hard — but smart — and progress will follow.

Section 5:
Weekly Split Examples

Now that we've covered training techniques, rep ranges, and intensity guidelines, it's time to see how they fit into full workout schedules. Below are three of the most common and effective splits: the **3-day full-body split**, the **4-day upper/lower split**, and the **5-day body-part emphasis split**. Each comes with its own strengths and trade-offs, making them suitable for different lifestyles, goals, and levels of experience.

The 3-Day Split (Balanced Full-Body Focus)

Who it's for: Beginners, busy professionals, or anyone who only has three days per week to train but still wants to build strength and size.

Structure:

Monday – Strength (Compounds + Progressive Overload)
Wednesday – Hypertrophy (Isolation + Drop Sets)
Friday – Conditioning & Joint Health (TriCon + Circuits)

Day-by-Day Breakdown:

Day 1 – Strength

Squat → 5×5 (heavy, progressive overload)
Bench Press → 5×5
Pull-Ups (weighted if possible) → 4×6–8
Overhead Press → 4×8

Focus: Low reps, heavy compound lifts, long rest (2–3 min).

Day 2 – Hypertrophy

Incline Dumbbell Press → 4×10–12 (last set drop)
Lateral Raises → 3×12–15
Leg Extensions → 4×12–15 (last set drop)
Barbell or Cable Curl → 3×10–12 (tempo slow eccentrics)

Focus: Moderate weights, controlled reps, pump-driven accessory work.

Day 3 – Conditioning/TriCon

Romanian Deadlifts (TriCon: 3 explosive, 3 hold, 3 slow) → 3×9
Circuit: Push-Ups → Goblet Squats → Inverted Rows → 3–5
rounds
Core Finisher: Planks & Side Planks → 3×45–60s

Focus: Joint-friendly training, higher reps, short rests (30–60s).

Why It Works:
Every muscle is trained multiple times per week without over-whelming recovery. The mix of strength, hypertrophy, and conditioning creates a balanced foundation.

The 4-Day Split (Upper/Lower Emphasis)

Who it's for: Intermediates who want more volume per muscle group and can commit to four training days weekly.

Structure:

Monday – Upper Strength (Compounds)
Tuesday – Lower Strength (Pyramids)
Thursday – Upper Hypertrophy (Isolation + Drop Sets)
Friday – Lower Conditioning (HIT + TriCon)

Day-by-Day Breakdown:

Day 1 – Upper Strength

Bench Press → 5×5
Barbell Row → 5×5
Overhead Press → 4×6–8
Weighted Dips → 3×8–10

Focus: Heavy compound lifts, pushing and pulling strength.

Day 2 – Lower Strength

Back Squat (pyramid: 12–10–8–6–4)
Deadlift (pyramid: 10–8–6–4)

Walking Lunges → 3×10–12/leg
Standing Calf Raises → 4×15 (tempo-controlled)

Focus: Strength and endurance blend, heavy pyramids for progression.

Day 3 – Upper Hypertrophy

Incline Dumbbell Press → 4×10–12
Lateral Raises → 4×12–15 (last set drop)
Lat Pulldown or Cable Row → 3×10–12
Barbell Curl (tempo slow eccentrics) → 3×12
Rope Triceps Pushdowns → 3×12–15

Focus: Moderate weight, high volume, pump work.

Day 4 – Lower Conditioning

Goblet Squats → 3–4×15
Step-Ups → 3×12/leg
Romanian Deadlifts (TriCon style) → 3×9
Core Circuit: Hanging Leg Raises → Russian Twists → Side Plank (3 rounds)

Focus: Conditioning, core work, joint-friendly TriCon.

Why It Works:
Each muscle group is trained twice weekly — once heavy, once lighter/higher rep — striking a balance between strength and hypertrophy. Recovery is manageable because upper and lower body alternate.

The 5-Day Split (Body-Part Emphasis)

Who it's for: Advanced trainees who want maximum hypertrophy, aesthetics, and specialization. Requires strong recovery and 5+ available days.

Structure:

Monday – Chest/Triceps (Drop Sets + Tempo)
Tuesday – Back/Biceps (Compounds + Isolation)

Wednesday – Legs (Pyramid + HIT
Thursday – Shoulders/Abs (Isolation + Tempo)
Friday – Full Body Conditioning (Supersets + Circuits)

Day-by-Day Breakdown:

Day 1 – Chest/Triceps

Bench Press → 5×5
Incline Dumbbell Press → 4×10–12 (drop set finisher)
Dips (slow descent) → 3×8
Rope Pushdowns → 3×12–15

Focus: Chest and triceps hypertrophy with intensity techniques.

Day 2 – Back/Biceps

Pull-Ups → 4×6–8
Barbell Row → 4×8–10
Lat Pulldown → 3×10–12
Dumbbell Curls → 3×12 (tempo-controlled)

Focus: Vertical and horizontal pulls, bicep isolation.

Day 3 – Legs

Back Squat (pyramid 12–10–8–6–4)
Romanian Deadlifts → 4×10
Leg Press → 3×12–15 (drop set finisher)
Walking Lunges → 3×12/leg

Focus: Heavy pyramids plus high-rep finishers for growth.

Day 4 – Shoulders/Abs

Overhead Press → 4×8
Lateral Raises (tempo 3–1–3) → 4×12–15
Rear Delt Fly → 3×12
Ab Circuit: Hanging Leg Raises → Cable Crunch → Plank (3 rounds)

Focus: Shoulder development and core strength.

Day 5 – Full Body Conditioning

Superset: Push-Ups + Pull-Ups (4 rounds, 10 reps each)
Superset: Squats + Romanian Deadlifts (4 rounds, 12 reps each)
Circuit Finisher: Burpees → Kettlebell Swings → Sit-Ups (3 rounds, 12 reps each)

Focus: High-density training for conditioning and calorie burn.

Why It Works:

This split allows maximum focus on each muscle group while keeping a day for conditioning. It's excellent for physique development but requires strong recovery and consistent effort.

Key Comparison

3-Day Split: Best for beginners, busy people, or those wanting balance.
4-Day Split: Great for intermediates who want more frequency and volume.
5-Day Split: Best for advanced lifters chasing hypertrophy and specialization.

Bottom Line: These examples are templates, not rules. You can substitute exercises based on available equipment or personal preference. What matters most is applying **progressive overload**, maintaining **consistency**, and respecting **recovery**.

Section 6:
Sample Workouts

The following programs are designed to match the splits outlined earlier. Each includes **compound lifts for strength**, **isolation moves for hypertrophy**, and **conditioning/core elements** for balance. Effort guidelines (RPE/RIR) are included to help you train hard but smart.

3-Day Split (Balanced Full-Body Focus)

Day 1 – Strength (Compounds + Progressive Overload)

Back Squat → 5×5 @ RPE 7–8 (2–3 RIR), rest 2–3 min
Bench Press → 5×5 @ RPE 7–8, rest 2–3 min
Pull-Ups (weighted if possible) → 4×6–8 @ RPE 8, rest 2–3 min
Overhead Press → 4×8 @ RPE 8, rest 90s–2 min
Optional Accessory: Barbell Hip Thrust or Row → 3×8–10

Day 2 – Hypertrophy (Isolation + Drop Sets)

Incline Dumbbell Press → 4×10–12 (last set drop 20–25%), RPE 8–9, rest 60–90s
Lateral Raises → 4×12–15 (slow tempo 2–1–2), rest 60s
Leg Extensions → 4×12–15 (last set drop), RPE 9, rest 60–90s
Barbell or Cable Curl → 3×10–12 (eccentric 3–1–3), RPE 8, rest 60s
Rope Pushdowns → 3×12–15, RPE 8, rest 60s

Day 3 – Conditioning / TriCon

Romanian Deadlift (TriCon: 3 explosive + 3 isometric + 3 slow) → 3–4×9, rest 90–120s
Circuit (3–5 rounds, 30–45s rest between moves):
Push-Ups ×12
Goblet Squats ×12
Inverted Rows ×10
Core Finisher: Plank (front & side) → 3×45–60s

4-Day Split (Upper/Lower)

Day 1 – Upper Strength (Compounds)

Bench Press → 5×5 @ RPE 7–8, rest 2–3 min

Barbell Row → 5×5, rest 2–3 min
Overhead Press → 4×6–8, rest 2 min
Weighted Dips → 3×8–10, rest 90s
Optional Accessory: Face Pulls → 3×12–15

Day 2 – Lower Strength (Pyramids)

Back Squat → 5 sets (12–10–8–6–4), rest 2–3 min
Deadlift → 4 sets (10–8–6–4), rest 2–3 min
Walking Lunges → 3×12/leg, rest 90s
Standing Calf Raises → 4×15 (tempo 2–1–2), rest 60–90s

Day 3 – Upper Hypertrophy (Isolation + Drop Sets)

Incline Dumbbell Press → 4×10–12 (last set drop), rest 60–90s
Lateral Raises → 4×12–15 (last set drop), rest 60s
Cable Row or Lat Pulldown → 3×10–12, rest 60–90s
Barbell Curl → 3×10–12 (slow eccentric), rest 60s
Rope Pushdowns → 3×12–15, rest 60s

Day 4 – Lower Conditioning (HIT + TriCon)

Goblet Squat → 3–4×15, rest 60–90s
Step-Ups → 3×12/leg, rest 60s
Romanian Deadlift (TriCon style) → 3×9, rest 90s
Core Circuit (3 rounds, short rest):
Hanging Leg Raises ×12
Russian Twists ×15/side
Side Plank ×30–45s

5-Day Split (Body-Part Emphasis)

Day 1 – Chest/Triceps (Drop Sets + Tempo)

Bench Press → 5×5, rest 2–3 min
Incline Dumbbell Press → 4×10–12 (last set drop), rest 90s
Dips (tempo: slow 3s descent) → 3×8–10, rest 90s
Rope Pushdowns → 3–4×12–15, rest 60s

Day 2 – Back/Biceps

Pull-Ups → 4×6–8, rest 2–3 min
Barbell Row → 4×8–10, rest 2–3 min
Lat Pulldown → 3×10–12, rest 60–90s
Dumbbell Curl (tempo: slow eccentric) → 3×12, rest 60s

Day 3 – Legs (Pyramid + HIT)

Back Squat (pyramid 12–10–8–6–4), rest 2–3 min
Romanian Deadlift → 4×10, rest 2 min
Leg Press → 3×12–15 (last set drop), rest 90s
Walking Lunges → 3×12/leg, rest 90s

Day 4 – Shoulders/Abs (Isolation + Tempo)

Overhead Press → 4×6–8, rest 2 min
Lateral Raises (tempo 2–1–2) → 4×12–15, rest 60s
Rear Delt Fly → 3×12, rest 60s
Core Giant Set (3–4 rounds, minimal rest):
Hanging Leg Raise ×12
Cable Crunch ×15
Plank ×45s

Day 5 – Full Body Conditioning (Supersets + Circuits)

Superset A: Push-Ups ×12 + Pull-Ups ×6–10 → 4 rounds, rest 60s
Superset B: Front Squat ×8–10 + Romanian Deadlift ×10–12 → 4 rounds, rest 90s
Circuit Finisher (3 rounds, short rest):
Burpees ×12
Kettlebell Swings ×15
Sit-Ups ×15

Key Notes on Using These Workouts

Warm-Up: Always include 5–10 minutes of mobility and light cardio before lifting, plus warm-up sets for main lifts.

Progression: Track weights and reps. Add weight once you can hit the top of the rep range with good form at the prescribed RPE.

Substitutions: If you lack equipment (e.g., no barbell), swap with a dumbbell or bodyweight variation. Example: DB rows instead of barbell rows.

De-loads: Every 6–8 weeks, reduce volume by ~30% to allow recovery before ramping intensity back up.

Bottom Line: These are complete, ready-to-use programs that blend strength, hypertrophy, and conditioning into structured weekly splits. By following the rep ranges, RPE/RIR guidelines, and progression strategies, you'll avoid plateaus and steadily improve over 12 weeks and beyond.

This Page Is Left Blank Intentionally

Section 7:
The 12 Week Progression System

One of the most important principles in strength training and physique development is **progression** — the idea that your body adapts when you gradually increase the demands placed upon it. Without structured progression, even the best-designed workout will stop producing results after a few weeks. The **12-week progression system** outlined here is designed to give you a **clear roadmap**, ensuring steady gains in strength, muscle growth (hypertrophy), and conditioning while avoiding burnout or injury.

This system is divided into three distinct phases:

Foundation (Weeks 1–4) – Learn, adapt, and set a baseline.

Growth (Weeks 5–8) – Increase training volume and stimulate hypertrophy.

Intensity (Weeks 9–12) – Push strength and conditioning close to your limits.

After these 12 weeks, you can take a **De-load week** (a lighter training week for recovery) before repeating or advancing the cycle.

Why Structured Phases Matter

Your muscles, connective tissues, and nervous system don't all adapt at the same pace. For example:

Muscles respond relatively quickly to training stress.

Tendons and ligaments adapt more slowly.

The nervous system (how your brain communicates with your muscles) adapts fastest but can also fatigue fastest.

By **cycling intensity and volume** (the amount of work you do), you allow all systems to progress together. This prevents overuse injuries and maximizes long-term results.

Understanding Training Variables

Before diving into the week-by-week plan, here are key terms we'll reference throughout:

Sets and Reps (Repetitions): A set is a group of reps performed without rest. Example: 3×10 means 3 sets of 10 reps.

Volume: The total work performed (sets × reps × weight). Higher volume usually stimulates more hypertrophy.

Intensity: How heavy the load is relative to your maximum. Often measured by **RPE (Rate of Perceived Exertion)** or **RIR (Reps in Reserve).**

RPE: A scale from 1–10 describing how hard a set feels. RPE 10 = all-out effort, no reps left; RPE 7 = you could do 3 more reps.

RIR: A measure of how many reps you had "left in the tank." RIR 2 = you could have done two more reps before failure.

Progressive Overload: The gradual increase of training stress (heavier weights, more reps, shorter rest, or added sets).

Phase 1: Foundation (Weeks 1–4)

Objective: Build consistency, perfect technique, and prepare your body for heavier loads.

Load (Weight Used): Light-to-moderate, around **RPE 6–7** (meaning 3–4 RIR).

Volume: 8–12 total sets per muscle group per week.

Reps: Stick to the lower-to-middle end of rep ranges. **Example:** 6–8 reps for compound lifts, 8–10 reps for isolation lifts.

Rest Between Sets: 90–120 seconds for most lifts, 2–3 minutes for heavy compounds.

Guidelines:

Focus on **form over weight.** Every rep should be crisp and repeatable.

Use this phase to **learn movement patterns**: squat, hinge (deadlift pattern), push, pull, and carry.

Keep logs: record weights, reps, and how hard the set felt (RPE).

Avoid going to failure — always leave 2–4 reps in reserve.

Week-by-Week:

Week 1: Establish baseline weights (choose weights that feel moderately challenging).

Week 2: Repeat with slightly smoother form and perhaps an extra rep on one exercise.

Week 3: Increase weight by 2.5–5 lbs on upper-body lifts (bench press, overhead press, rows) and 5–10 lbs on lower-body lifts (squats, deadlifts).

Week 4: Add one additional rep per set if possible, maintaining form.

Why It Matters: This phase creates a safe "training base." It strengthens tendons and ligaments, builds coordination, and sets habits that prevent injury when training intensifies later.

Phase 2: Growth (Weeks 5–8)

Objective: Push training volume higher to stimulate hypertrophy (muscle growth).

Load: Moderate-to-heavy, around **RPE 7–8** (2–3 RIR).

Volume: 12–15 sets per muscle group per week.

Reps: Hypertrophy-focused (8–12 reps for compound lifts, 10–15 reps for isolation).

Rest: 60–90 seconds for accessory lifts, 2 minutes for heavy compounds.

Guidelines:

Start **progressive overload**: aim to add weight or reps each week.

Add one **extra set** for muscle groups you want to prioritize (e.g., chest, legs, back).

Introduce advanced techniques **sparingly**:

Drop Sets: After finishing a set, immediately reduce the weight by 20–30% and continue until near failure.

Tempo Training: Slow down the lowering phase (eccentric) to increase time under tension.

TriCon Training (Triple Contraction): 3 explosive reps, 3 isometric holds, 3 slow reps — great for joint-friendly intensity.

Maintain **1–2 reps in reserve** for most lifts.

Week-by-Week:

Week 5: Increase loads by ~5% compared to Foundation phase.

Week 6: Keep weight stable but add a set on key lifts.

Week 7: Introduce drop sets for 2–3 accessory lifts.

Week 8: Push reps toward the higher end of the range (10–12 on compounds, 12–15 on isolation).

Why It Matters: This is the "workhorse" phase. The combination of higher volume and moderate-to-heavy intensity is the sweet spot for hypertrophy. Most muscle growth occurs here.

Phase 3: Intensity (Weeks 9–12)

Objective: Maximize strength and push muscles near their limits while slightly reducing volume to allow recovery.

Load: Heavy, around **RPE 8–9** (1–2 RIR, sometimes to failure on isolation work).

Volume: Moderate (10–12 sets per muscle per week).

Reps: Strength-focused (3–6 for big lifts, 6–10 for accessories).

Rest: 2–4 minutes for compounds, 60–90 seconds for isolation.

Guidelines:

Main compound lifts (squat, bench press, deadlift, overhead press) move to lower rep ranges with heavier loads.

Hypertrophy lifts stay in the 8–12 range, but you should push closer to failure (RPE 9–10).

Conditioning (circuits, high-intensity interval training, TriCon) is intensified with shorter rests and higher density.

Consider using **Rest-Pause Sets** (perform reps to near failure, rest 20–30 seconds, then continue) or **Cluster Sets** (breaking a set into smaller mini-sets with short rests).

Week-by-Week:

Week 9: Add 2.5–5 lbs to upper lifts, 5–10 lbs to lower lifts.

Week 10: Drop reps slightly on compounds (e.g., from 6 to 4), keeping load heavy.

Week 11: Push hypertrophy lifts closer to failure on the last set (RPE 9–10).

Week 12: Test your progress with rep personal records (PRs). Example: If you lifted 135 lbs for 8 reps in Week 4, aim for 145 lbs for 8 reps now.

Why It Matters: This phase emphasizes **intensity over volume**. You're teaching your body to handle heavier weights safely, while muscles adapt to maximum tension. It also reveals just how much progress you've made.

The De-load (Week 13 – Optional)

After 12 weeks, it's wise to take a **De-load week** before restarting the cycle.

Volume: Cut total sets in half.

Load: Drop weights to ~RPE 5–6 (4–5 RIR).

Focus: Technique practice, mobility, and recovery.

Why It Matters: Think of de-loads as maintenance for your body. They allow connective tissues to heal, restore nervous system energy, and ensure you can continue progressing long-term.

Applying Progression to Different Splits

3-Day Full-Body Split:

Weeks 1–4: Focus on form and consistent load.

Weeks 5–8: Add accessory volume and drop sets.

Weeks 9–12: Push heavier weights on squats, bench, and deadlifts while circuits become denser.

4-Day Upper/Lower Split:

Weeks 1–4: Establish rhythm and base strength.

Weeks 5–8: Increase accessory isolation work for arms and shoulders.

Weeks 9–12: Heavy compounds (squat, bench) prioritized; conditioning day becomes more demanding.

5-Day Body-Part Split:

Weeks 1–4: Leave 3–4 RIR (don't go to failure yet).

Weeks 5–8: Push volume higher with extra sets and techniques.

Weeks 9–12: Specialize — chest, legs, and back days get heavy;

arms and shoulders push close to failure.

Tracking and Measuring Results

To ensure you're progressing, track these markers:

Strength: Record weights and reps on core lifts. Compare Week 1 to Week 12.

RPE/RIR: Write down how hard sets felt to spot trends in fatigue or progress.

Visual Progress: Take photos every 4 weeks to see changes in muscle definition.

Recovery: Monitor sleep, soreness, and motivation. Declining performance signals the need for adjustment.

Bottom Line: The 12-week progression system is your **blueprint for sustainable success**. You begin by learning and adapting, then build muscle through higher volume, and finally peak by pushing intensity. With a De-load, you're ready to restart the cycle stronger and fitter than before.

Section 8:
Home & Minimal Equipment Adaptations

Not everyone has access to a fully equipped gym, and even seasoned lifters sometimes face seasons where training has to be done at home or on the road. The good news is that the principles of **progressive overload** (gradually increasing the challenge over time), **training splits** (how you divide workouts across the week), and the **12-week progression system** still apply. You simply have to choose exercises that fit your environment.

This section will show you how to adapt the **3-day, 4-day, and 5-day splits** to a **minimal equipment setup**, using:

Bodyweight (push-ups, pull-ups, lunges).

Resistance bands (rows, presses, extensions).

Dumbbells or kettlebells (squats, presses, carries).

Household items (backpacks loaded with books, water jugs, sturdy chairs).

Key Adaptation Principles

Rep Ranges Expand at Home

In the gym, hypertrophy is often trained at **6–12 reps**. At home, with lighter loads, you may need to push to **15–30 reps per set**, especially with bodyweight or bands.

Hypertrophy still happens as long as you train near failure (0–3 RIR).

Tempo Control is Your Best Friend

Slow down the eccentric (lowering phase) to increase time under tension. **Example:** push-ups with a 3–4 second descent.

Pauses at the bottom or isometric holds (TriCon style) make light weights feel heavy.

Circuits Save Time and Increase Density

When equipment is limited, pairing movements back-to-back

(supersets or circuits) increases training stress without needing heavier weights.

Progression Still Matters

Add reps, add sets, shorten rest, slow the tempo, or increase resistance (heavier bands, backpack loading) to apply progressive overload.

Example Adaptations by Split

3-Day Split (Full-Body, Minimal Equipment)

Day 1 – Strength Focus

Backpack Squats → 4×12–15
Push-Ups (weighted if possible) → 4×12–20
Inverted Rows (under a sturdy table) → 4×10–12
Pike Press (shoulder focus) → 3×8–12

Day 2 – Hypertrophy Focus

Bulgarian Split Squats (bodyweight or holding dumbbells) → 4×12/leg
Banded Chest Press → 4×12–15
Banded Rows → 4×12–15
Biceps Curl with Bands or Dumbbells → 3×12–15

Day 3 – Conditioning / Core

Circuit (3–5 rounds, 30s rest):
Jump Squats ×15
Push-Ups ×15
Mountain Climbers ×20/side
Core Finisher: Side Planks 3×30–60s per side

4-Day Split (Upper/Lower at Home)

Day 1 – Upper Strength

Pike Push-Ups (shoulder emphasis) → 4×8–12

Banded Rows → 4×12–15
Backpack Floor Press → 4×10–12
Chin-Ups (doorframe bar) → 3×max reps

Day 2 – Lower Strength

Bulgarian Split Squats → 4×12–15
Backpack Deadlifts → 4×12
Banded Good Mornings → 3×15
Calf Raises (on stairs) → 4×20

Day 3 – Upper Hypertrophy

Diamond Push-Ups → 3×12–20
Banded Lateral Raises → 3×15–20
Backpack Rows (tempo-controlled) → 4×10–12
Band Face Pulls → 3×15–20

Day 4 – Lower Conditioning

Walking Lunges (bodyweight or holding dumbbells) → 4×20 steps
Jump Squats → 3×12
Glute Bridges (banded or weighted with backpack) → 4×15
Core Circuit: Bicycle Crunches ×20/side → Side Planks ×30–60s → Repeat 3 rounds

5-Day Split (Body-Part Emphasis, Home Version)

Day 1 – Chest/Triceps

Push-Ups (weighted or tempo) → 5×12–20
Banded Chest Fly → 3×12–15
Dips (between chairs) → 4×10–12
Banded Triceps Pushdowns → 3×15

Day 2 – Back/Biceps

Pull-Ups or Inverted Rows → 5×max reps
Banded Rows → 4×12–15
Dumbbell or Banded Curls → 3×12–15

Backpack Shrugs → 3×20

Day 3 – Legs

Bulgarian Split Squats → 4×12/leg
Backpack Squats → 4×12–15
Banded Good Mornings → 3×15
Jump Squats → 3×12

Day 4 – Shoulders/Abs

Pike Push-Ups → 4×8–12
Banded Lateral Raises → 4×15–20
Rear Delt Rows (bands or light dumbbells) → 3×15
Core Circuit: Hanging Leg Raises ×12 → Russian Twists ×20 →
Plank ×45s

Day 5 – Conditioning

Circuit (4–5 rounds, minimal rest):
Burpees ×12
Jump Lunges ×12/leg
Push-Ups ×15
Mountain Climbers ×20/side

Progression at Home (Weeks 1–12)

Weeks 1–4 (Foundation): Focus on control and consistency. Start with lower reps if needed (8–12), but build toward higher ranges (15–20).

Weeks 5–8 (Growth): Add sets, reduce rest, and include pauses or tempo variations. Example: 3-second descent on push-ups.

Weeks 9–12 (Intensity): Push to near failure (RPE 9–10, meaning no reps left in reserve) on bodyweight and banded moves. Add extra circuit rounds for conditioning.

Advantages of Minimal Equipment Training

Accessibility: You can train anywhere, anytime.

Joint-Friendly: Lighter loads with bands and bodyweight reduce wear and tear.

Functional Strength: Many at-home moves mimic real-life activities (carrying, pushing, pulling).

Progression Still Works: As long as you increase the challenge, the body adapts — regardless of whether you use a barbell or a backpack.

Bottom Line: Home and minimal equipment training is not a watered-down version of gym training. By applying progressive overload with reps, sets, tempo, and circuits, you can achieve **remarkable strength, hypertrophy, and conditioning results** even without traditional gym equipment.

Section 9:
Recovery, Nutrition, and Lifestyle Integration

Most people think results come solely from the workouts themselves. In reality, the **stimulus happens in the gym, but the adaptations — strength, muscle growth, fat loss, and improved conditioning — happen outside the gym** when your body recovers. Recovery and nutrition are the "other half" of training. Without them, even the best 12-week program stalls.

This section covers:

Recovery Fundamentals – sleep, rest days, stress management.

Nutrition for Training – macro-nutrients, meal timing, hydration, supplements.

Lifestyle Integration – habits, consistency, and balancing training with real life.

Recovery Fundamentals

Sleep: The Master Recovery Tool

Aim for **7–9 hours of sleep per night**.

Growth hormone (GH) and testosterone, two key anabolic (muscle-building) hormones, spike during deep sleep.

Poor sleep impairs strength, slows muscle recovery, and increases fat storage.

Sleep Hygiene Tips:

Keep a consistent bedtime and wake time (even on weekends).

Avoid screens 30–60 minutes before bed — blue light delays melatonin release.

Keep your bedroom dark, cool, and quiet.

Try a pre-bed routine: stretching, reading, or journaling.

Rest Days: When You Grow

Rest days are not "lost days" — they're when your body repairs muscle fibers and restores energy.

At least **1–2 rest days per week** are recommended, depending on your split.

Active recovery (light walking, yoga, mobility work) is better than complete inactivity.

Stress Management

Training is a form of **stress**. Add work, family, or financial stress, and the body can tip into recovery debt.

High stress raises cortisol (a catabolic hormone), which can interfere with muscle gain and fat loss.

Practical tools: daily walks, breathwork, meditation, or even unplugging from social media before bed.

Nutrition for Training

Nutrition fuels performance and recovery. Think of it as **building a house**:

Training is the blueprint (stimulus).

Nutrition is the bricks, cement, and tools (raw materials).

Macro-nutrients: The Big 3

1. Protein – *The builder*

Role: Muscle repair, recovery, growth.

Target: **1.6–2.2 grams per kilogram of bodyweight** (or ~0.7–1.0 g per pound).

Sources: Lean meats, poultry, fish, eggs, dairy, legumes, whey or plant protein powders.

Distribution: Spread protein intake evenly across **3–5 meals/**

snacks per day, each with 20–40 g protein.

2. Carbohydrates (Carbs) – *The fuel*

Role: Primary energy source for resistance training and high-intensity exercise.

Target: **3–6 g per kilogram of bodyweight** depending on training volume.

Sources: Rice, oats, potatoes, fruit, vegetables, whole grains.

Timing: Consume carbs **before and after training** to fuel and replenish glycogen (stored energy).

3. Fats – *The regulator*

Role: Hormone production (including testosterone), joint health, energy.

Target: **~20–30% of daily calories**.

Sources: Nuts, seeds, olive oil, avocados, fatty fish.

Meal Timing: When to Eat

Pre-Workout (1–3 hours before):

Balanced meal of carbs + protein, low in fat.

Example: Chicken, rice, and vegetables.

Intra-Workout:

Not necessary for most unless training 90+ minutes.

A sports drink or small carb snack can help if needed.

Post-Workout (within 2 hours):

Carbs + protein are key for recovery.

Example: Whey protein shake + banana.

Hydration

Dehydration of just **2% bodyweight** can reduce performance.

Target: **30–40 mL per kg bodyweight per day** (~2.5–3.5 liters for most).

Electrolytes matter if training hard in heat or sweating heavily.

Signs you're under-hydrated: dark urine, low energy, frequent cramps.

Supplements (Optional but Helpful)

Evidence-backed supplements include:

Creatine Monohydrate: 5 g/day, supports strength, hypertrophy, and recovery.

Whey Protein: Convenient source of high-quality protein.

Caffeine: 3–6 mg per kg bodyweight pre-workout can boost strength and focus.

Fish Oil (Omega-3s): Anti-inflammatory benefits, supports joint and heart health.

Multivitamin: Fills dietary gaps, especially in restrictive diets.

Lifestyle Integration

Consistency Beats Perfection

Missing a workout or having a less-than-perfect meal won't ruin progress. What matters is the **average over weeks and months**.

Aim for **80/20 balance**: 80% whole, nutrient-dense foods and consistent training; 20% flexibility for life's realities.

Daily Habits That Compound Results

Walking 7,000–10,000 steps/day improves recovery and cardiovascular health.

Stretching or mobility drills for 5–10 minutes daily prevent stiffness.

Meal prepping makes hitting protein and calorie goals far easier.

Logging workouts keeps you accountable and shows objective progress.

Balancing Training With Real Life

Choose a split that fits your schedule. If you can realistically train 3 days/week, a 3-day split done consistently beats a 5-day plan you can't stick to.

Travel or work stress? Swap a heavy session for bodyweight circuits.

Kids at home? Involve them in active recovery days (walks, bike rides, playing outside).

Integrating Recovery, Nutrition, and Training

The 12-week progression system only works if recovery and nutrition keep pace. Think of the triangle:

Training → provides the stimulus.

Nutrition → provides the building blocks.

Recovery → allows adaptation to occur.

If one side of the triangle is missing, progress slows or stalls.

Example:

Training hard but sleeping 5 hours/night? Expect stalled lifts and poor recovery.

Eating enough protein but skipping carbs? Energy will tank, and progress will slow.

Resting plenty but not applying progressive overload? No stimulus = no growth.

Bottom Line: Recovery, nutrition, and lifestyle habits are not "extras" — they are the foundation of progress. Lift with intent, eat with purpose, and rest with discipline. When training, nutrition, and recovery align, you create the conditions for consistent strength, hypertrophy, and lifelong health.

This Page is Left Blank Intentionally

Section 10:
Putting It All Together
(The Integrated Roadmap)

By now, you've learned about **workout splits, training techniques, progression systems, recovery, and nutrition.** Each piece is powerful on its own, but the real transformation happens when they are combined into one integrated plan. This section acts as your **roadmap** — showing you how to take all the moving parts and turn them into a daily, weekly, and long-term system you can live by.

Step 1: Choose Your Split

3-Day Split: Best for beginners, busy schedules, or those wanting balance with recovery.

4-Day Split: Ideal for intermediates who want more frequency and volume.

5-Day Split: Best for advanced trainees who can recover from higher intensity and want specialization.

Pick the split that fits your **schedule and lifestyle**, not the one that looks hardest on paper. Consistency matters most.

Step 2: Apply the 12-Week Progression System

Every split follows the **Foundation → Growth → Intensity** cycle:

Weeks 1–4 (Foundation): Learn form, build consistency, and establish baseline weights.

Weeks 5–8 (Growth): Add sets, push volume, introduce advanced techniques (drop sets, tempo, TriCon).

Weeks 9–12 (Intensity): Push near your limits with heavier weights, lower reps, and advanced methods like rest-pause or cluster sets.

Week 13 (Optional De-load): Reduce volume and intensity to recover fully before restarting.

Whether at home or in the gym, this structure ensures steady, measurable gains.

Step 3: Use Global Guidelines for Sets, Reps, and Effort

Strength: 3–6 reps per set, heavy loads, longer rest (2–4 minutes).

Hypertrophy: 6–12 reps (or up to 20–30 with light loads near failure), moderate rests (60–90 seconds).

Endurance/Conditioning: 12–20+ reps, short rests (30–60 seconds), circuits or supersets.

Effort: Train to within **1–3 reps in reserve (RIR)** most of the time. Push to **RPE 9–10 (all-out effort)** sparingly.

Step 4: Prioritize Recovery

Sleep: 7–9 hours per night.

Rest Days: 1–2 per week with light activity (walking, stretching).

Stress Management: Keep cortisol in check with meditation, journaling, or nature walks.

De-load Weeks: Every 6–12 weeks depending on fatigue and performance.

Think of recovery as your **secret weapon** — it's where growth happens.

Step 5: Dial in Nutrition

Protein: 1.6–2.2 g per kg bodyweight daily (spread across 3–5 meals).

Carbohydrates: 3–6 g per kg bodyweight, focus around workouts for fuel and recovery.

Fats: 20–30% of total calories, emphasizing healthy sources (avocados, nuts, olive oil, fish).

Hydration: 2.5–3.5 liters per day, more if sweating heavily.

Supplements (Optional but Useful): Creatine (5 g/day), whey protein, caffeine, fish oil, multivitamin.

Step 6: Adapt to Environment

Gym Access: Use barbells, dumbbells, cables, and machines.

Minimal Equipment: Use bands, dumbbells, backpacks, and bodyweight.

Travel: Stick with bodyweight circuits and high-rep, near-failure training.

No matter your setting, the principles of **progressive overload, effort, and recovery** apply universally.

Step 7: Track and Reflect

Workout Log: Write down weights, sets, reps, and RPE (Rate of Perceived Exertion).

Photos & Measurements: Take progress photos and waist/hip/arm measurements every 4 weeks.

Recovery Log: Record sleep, soreness, and energy levels.

Adjustments: If performance stalls for 2–3 weeks, reduce volume or intensity, or schedule a De-load.

Step 8: Commit to the Long Game

Think in **cycles**, not single workouts. Every 12 weeks is a new opportunity to refine.

Small improvements (1 more rep, 2.5 lbs more weight, 5 seconds longer plank) compound over months and years.

Balance matters: Training is one piece of your life — let it enhance your health, energy, and confidence, not consume it.

The Roadmap in Practice
(A Sample Week – 4-Day Split, Growth Phase)

Day 1 (Upper – Strength Focus):
Bench Press 4×6 @ RPE 7
Bent-Over Rows 4×8
Overhead Press 3×8
Pull-Ups 3×AMRAP (as many reps as possible).

Day 2 (Lower – Hypertrophy Focus):
Squats 4×8
Romanian Deadlifts 3×10
Walking Lunges 3×12/leg
Calf Raises 4×20.

Day 3 (Upper – Hypertrophy Focus):
Incline Dumbbell Press 4×10
Lat Pulldowns 4×12
Lateral Raises 3×15
Face Pulls 3×15

Day 4 (Lower – Strength + Conditioning):
Deadlifts 4×5, Front
Squats 3×6, Step-Ups 3×12,
Circuit: Jump Squats + Plank + Burpees (3 rounds).

Day 5–7: Rest: *walking, stretching, or light cardio.*

This is just one example, but it illustrates how the **split, progression system, set/rep guidelines, recovery, and nutrition principles come together.**

Bottom Line: Training is not about guessing or following random workouts. It's about **systems and cycles** — choosing the right split, progressing week to week, eating to fuel performance, recovering deeply, and repeating the process. If you follow this roadmap with consistency, you will see measurable improvements in strength, muscle, and overall health within 12 weeks — and more importantly, you'll have built habits for a lifetime.

This Page is Left Blank Intentionally

Section 11:
12 Week Sample Progression Workout Plans

How to Use This Plans

1. Choose your split (3, 4, or 5 days per week). Stick to it consistently.

2. Follow the weekly workouts as written. Log your **weights, reps, and RPE/RIR** each session.

3. Progress each phase:

Weeks 1–4 (Foundation): Focus on form, moderate weights, consistency.

Weeks 5–8 (Growth): Increase volume, add drop sets, shorten rest slightly.

Weeks 9–12 (Intensity): Heavier loads, advanced techniques, peak effort.

4. Rest as prescribed:

Strength: 2–3 min
Hypertrophy: 60–90 sec
Conditioning/Accessory: 30–60 sec

3-Day Split (Full Body Balance)
Weekly Schedule

Mon: Strength (Compounds + Progressive Overload)
Wed: Hypertrophy (Isolation + Drop Sets)
Fri: Conditioning (TriCon + Circuits)

Weeks 1–4 (Foundation)

Day 1 (Strength)

Squat – 4×5
Bench Press – 4×5
Pull-Ups (assisted/weighted) – 4×6–8
Overhead Press – 3×8

Day 2 (Hypertrophy)

Incline Dumbbell Press – 3×10–12
Lateral Raises – 3×12–15
Leg Extensions – 3×12
Barbell Curl – 3×10–12

Day 3 (Conditioning)

Romanian Deadlifts (TriCon style) – 3×9
Circuit: Push-Ups → Bodyweight Squats → Inverted Rows – 3 rounds × 12 reps
Plank – 3×45 sec

Weeks 5–8 (Growth)

Add 1 set to each main lift.
Introduce drop sets on isolation (final set).
Conditioning circuits → 4 rounds, 45 sec rest.

Weeks 9–12 (Intensity)

Compounds: Push heavier 4×4–6.
Hypertrophy: Double drops on final set.
TriCon: Extend holds to 8–10 sec.
Circuits: 5 rounds, 30 sec rest.

4-Day Split (Upper/Lower) Weekly Schedule

Mon: Upper Strength
Tue: Lower Strength
Thu: Upper Hypertrophy
Fri: Lower Conditioning (HIT + TriCon)

Weeks 1–4 (Foundation)

Day 1 (Upper Strength)

Bench Press – 5×5
Barbell Row – 5×5

Overhead Press – 4×6–8
Dips – 3×8–10

Day 2 (Lower Strength)

Squat (pyramid 12–10–8–6–4)
Deadlift (pyramid 10–8–6–4)
Walking Lunges – 3×12/leg
Calf Raises – 4×15

Day 3 (Upper Hypertrophy)

Incline Dumbbell Press – 4×10–12
Lateral Raises – 3×15
Bicep Curl – 3×12 (tempo 3–1–3)
Rope Tricep Pushdowns – 3×12–15

Day 4 (Lower Conditioning)

Goblet Squats – 3×15
Step-Ups – 3×12/leg
Romanian Deadlifts (TriCon) – 3×9
Core Circuit: Hanging Leg Raises → Russian Twists → Side Plank
– 3 rounds

Weeks 5–8 (Growth)

Add 1 set to compounds.
Add drop sets to isolation.
Conditioning: 4 rounds, 45 sec rest.

Weeks 9–12 (Intensity)

Compounds: Top set heavy (RPE 9).
Hypertrophy: Double/triple drops on last set.
Conditioning: 5 rounds, 30 sec rest.

5-Day Split (Body-Part Focus)
Weekly Schedule

Mon: Chest/Triceps

Tue: Back/Biceps
Wed: Legs
Thu: Shoulders/Abs
Fri: Full-Body Conditioning

Weeks 1–4 (Foundation)

Day 1 (Chest/Triceps)

Bench Press – 5×5
Incline Dumbbell Press – 4×10
Dips – 3×8–10 (tempo slow descent)
Rope Pushdowns – 3×12

Day 2 (Back/Biceps)

Pull-Ups – 4×6–8
Barbell Row – 4×8–10
Lat Pulldown – 3×12
Dumbbell Curl – 3×12

Day 3 (Legs)

Squat (pyramid 12–10–8–6–4)
Romanian Deadlift – 4×8–10
Leg Press – 3×12
Walking Lunges – 3×12/leg

Day 4 (Shoulders/Abs)

Overhead Press – 4×6–8
Lateral Raises – 3×12–15
Rear Delt Fly – 3×12–15
Ab Circuit: Hanging Leg Raises → Cable Crunch → Plank – 3 rounds

Day 5 (Conditioning)

Superset: Push-Ups + Pull-Ups – 4×10 each
Superset: Squats + RDLs – 4×10 each
Finisher Circuit: Burpees → Kettlebell Swings → Sit-Ups – 3 rounds

Weeks 5–8 (Growth)

Add 1–2 sets to compounds.
Drop sets on isolation moves.
Circuits: 4 rounds, 45 sec rest.

Weeks 9–12 (Intensity)

Compounds: Heavy 4–6 reps, RPE 9.
Isolation: Triple drop sets.
Conditioning: 5 rounds, 30 sec rest.

www.ingramcontent.com/pod-product-compliance
Lightning Source LLC
Chambersburg PA
CBHW071347290326
41933CB00041B/3022